Surgeon on Call

A Day in the Barrel

b c harris

Table of Contents

I

PROLOGUE

On Tuesday morning, Dr. Jones is thinking about the surgical call he must take on Friday. In the surgeon's lounge, he pours a cup of coffee and stands casually with his left shoulder leaning against the wall. He holds the coffee cup in his right hand. His face is angular and unsullied by gravity or the weight that accumulates with age. He looks youthful except for his preternaturally white hair. An older woman might find him attractive, while a younger woman would describe him as self assured.

The surgeon's lounge is the operating room equivalent of a holding pen. It is there surgeons wait before and between cases while the operating room staff prepares for the next surgical procedure. In the lounge with Dr. Jones is an older surgeon. The older surgeon sprawls comfortably on a dingy floral couch that occupies one side of the room. His feet, the shoes covered in light blue disposable surgical booties, rest on a battered cocktail table positioned in front of the couch.

Dr. Jones reflects and says, "You know...I hate call."

"Really?" the other man says. "Sometimes I think I hate everything about my job but the pay."

"Yeah? I'm not that far gone yet."

"You're younger."

"What kills me is somewhere right now the patient I'm going to operate on at, say, oh dark thirty Saturday morning is getting sick and, for some unfathomable reason, waiting to come to the Emergency Department until Friday when I'm on call."

"Friday is your day in the barrel?" the older surgeon says. "Hah! If you think of patients coming to the Emergency Department as an ocean, Friday and Saturday night are high tide."

"That helps my mood," Dr. Jones says sarcastically.

The older man grimaces and tilts his head. "Yes, but—"

"Dr. Jones, ready for you in room two," a voice over the intercom blares.

Dr. Jones is divorced. He is the father of two children. Molly, his oldest child, is a high school sophomore. She recently obtained her driver's license and is excited to be driving her own car to and from school. Since she is an inexperienced driver, she still has a 9:00 p.m. driving curfew. She is thin and has straight brunette hair. She is moody, quick to smile, and as quick to pout. Her brother, David, is quiet, reserved for an adolescent. When boredom or some other lowly impulse strikes him, he taunts his mercurial sister. Since getting her license, Molly has become her brother's de facto chauffeur. She shuttles him to school and between their parents' houses.

Dr. Jones's house is a rust-colored brick two-story in a residential neighborhood of similar houses. Although he has joint custody of the children with the former Mrs. Jones, the children only stay with him every other weekend. The exigencies of being on call can make even this arrangement complicated.

II

MORNING

On Friday morning after waiting until he knows she will be getting ready for school, Dr. Jones texts Molly: "On call today. Your plans?"

She texts back: "Pick up David after school. Go to football game. At your house by 9."

He responds: "Good. Text later. Money on table for dinner in case I can't be there."

Dr. Jones receives his first page of the morning while he is in the shower. Although smartphones are supplanting pagers as the contact method of choice, Dr. Jones has both a pager and a phone nearby. He hears the page but unhurriedly finishes his shower. After drying off, he wraps a towel around himself and looks at the number displayed on the pager. *Hmm, 3879,* he muses. He recognizes the number of one of the hospital floors, which means the call is about an inpatient. Since the patient has already been admitted, the call is less likely to be an emergency. Dr. Jones, still damp from the shower, picks up the phone and dials the number.

"Fifth floor," a receptionist answers. "How may I help?"

"Marie." Dr. Jones recognizes her voice. "Someone paged me?"

"Oh, yes. Dr. Madruh admitted a patient last night he wants you to see."

"What's the diagnosis?"

"Says here high blood pressure and cellulitis arm. Rule out abscess."

"OK. Put the patient on my computer list. I'll see him. Has he eaten?"

"I'll let you talk to the nurse about that."

There is the sound of clicking, then silence followed by ringing.

After several rings, Dr. Jones hears, "This is Carolyn."

"Carolyn, this is Dr. Jones." She knows his voice, but he identifies himself to her anyway. "Do you have Dr. Madruh's patient admitted last night with an infected arm?"

"Yes. That is my patient," she says expectantly.

"Has he eaten yet?"

"He just finished breakfast." The reply seems innocent enough.

Blood rushes to Dr. Jones's face. His voice quivers.

"What did he have?"

"Bacon, eggs, toast, grits."

"Get everything away from him now!" Dr. Jones barks. "Even water. He should be NPO."

NPO is the medical acronym for the Latin phrase *nil per os* or "nothing by mouth." Dr. Jones has instantly surmised that if the patient has an abscess, a pocket of pus, in his arm, then the necessary drainage procedure will have to be delayed until the patient has had time to digest breakfast.

For solid foods, the gastric emptying time is eight hours. Dr. Jones knows his colleagues in the Anesthesia Department will certainly want to wait the full eight hours. Though inconvenient, this is a safe practice to minimize the risk of the patient inhaling stomach contents into his lungs during induction of anesthesia. The procedure, drainage of soft tissue abscess arm, which will take no more than thirty minutes operative time, will have to wait eight hours. Dr. Jones looks at the clock on his nightstand: 7:38 a.m. He won't be able to operate on this patient until nearly 4:00 p.m. In a gesture of frustration, Dr. Jones flips his cell phone on the bed. The phone bounces once on the bedspread, landing screen up.

Dr. Jones decides to see the patient with the possible abscess first, make rounds at that hospital, and then travel across town to the other hospital he covers and perform the gallbladder surgery that is scheduled there for 10:30 a.m.

When he gets to the main doctor's lounge, Dr. Jones opens his patient list on one of several PCs provided for that purpose. There is only one new patient on his list, Mr. Carpen. When he looks at the patient's record, he is pleased to see that Mr. Carpen is the patient he was paged about earlier. *At least it's not another consult.* The data in the computer reveals that during his stay in the Emergency Department, Mr. Carpen had an ultrasound performed on his left arm. The ultrasound is reported as showing a 2 x 2 cm fluid collection just above the antecubital fossa, the area of the arm near the elbow crease. The radiologist interpreted this fluid collection as a possible abscess.

Right, Dr. Jones thinks. He calls the operating room scheduling desk.

"Karen, I have a case for this afternoon. Drainage of abscess, left arm. Mr. Carpen, room 514. He ate breakfast. Let anesthesia know. I can work anytime they give the OK. You'll call me back? Thanks."

Dr. Jones goes to the fifth floor to examine Mr. Carpen, a formality. Mr. Carpen is a grizzled, fifty-two-year-old white male. He has a barrel-shaped trunk from which extend four beefy extremities. The left arm is swollen from just below the armpit to the wrist. An ellipse of redness extends above and below the antecubital fossa. At peak redness, the swelling suggests a lemon buried firmly beneath the skin. By way of examination, Dr. Jones lightly touches the swollen arm.

"Hey, whatcha doin'?" Mr. Carpen blurts. "That hurts!"

Dr. Jones cursorily introduces himself. "I'm Dr. Jones. Dr. Madruh asked me to see you. I'm going to be your surgeon. The pus in that arm has to be drained."

"Well, something better be done. Hurts like hell! I need more pain meds. I can't take this."

Unfazed, Dr. Jones ignores the outburst and says, "Tell me, how did this start?"

"Three days ago, I was doing metal work in my garage, and my arm got scratched. Then it started swelling up."

"OK, I'm going to ask some questions while I examine you."

Dr. Jones moves about the patient, listening to the patient's heart and lungs with his stethoscope, watching how the patient moves his extremities, and asking questions all simultaneously.

"Do you use tobacco?"

"Smoke? Yeah. Pack or two a day."

"How about alcohol?" Dr. Jones leads the patient. "Six-pack per day? Per week?"

"I don't drink now. Used to."

"What about other drugs?"

"No," Mr. Carpen answers sullenly.

"You have an abscess—pus—in your arm that needs to be drained," Dr. Jones says. "Since you've eaten breakfast, surgery will be later this afternoon. We'll put you to sleep for about thirty minutes. There'll be a big, open wound on your arm from where I drain the pus. After surgery, you'll need dressing changes. We can talk about that later."

"OK, Doc. But what about pain? I need something for the pain."

"I'll see what Dr. Madruh ordered for you. I'm sure you have some pain medicine ordered."

"Yeah. It's not working. That's the problem!"

"It will be hard to get the pain to stop until I get the pus out. That will help a lot," Dr. Jones reassures the patient.

The interview and examination have been a bit of charade. There aren't any scratches on the patient's left arm. Deep soft tissue abscesses of the upper extremity are common in only a few clinical situations. Dr. Jones applies a simple diagnostic maxim from medical school: when you hear hoof beats, think of horses. The maxim means that the first diagnosis that comes to mind that explains a patient's presentation is likely to be correct. The sound of hoof beats, while conceivably caused by other animals, is most commonly caused by horses.

The patient, Mr. Carpen, is an intravenous drug user. Venipuncture using poor sterile technique, dirty needles, caustic drugs or a witches' brew of all three caused the arm infection.

Dr. Jones looks at his patient list and sees, as usual, that his patients are dispersed throughout the hospital. He estimates he has time to visit two uncomplicated postoperative patients before rushing to the other hospital. He finds the chart for the first patient and transcribes objective data (vital signs, urine output) into his notes. While he is examining the patient, his pager goes off. He recognizes the number, 909-2377, as the number of the operating room at the hospital across town where he will soon be headed.

"Excuse me," he tells the patient. "I have to answer this page." He steps away from the patient's bedside. With his back turned to the patient, he makes the call on his cell phone.

"Dr. Jones. You paged?" The tone of his voice is flat, monotone.

"Oh, Dr. Jones, will you be on time for your ten-thirty case?" the receptionist says cheerily.

"Yes. Plan to be." His reply is abrupt.

"OK. Good. Just checking."

The conversation over, Dr. Jones puts the cell phone back in his jacket pocket.

"Sorry," he says to the patient. "Now let's take a look at that wound."

With one hand, he draws down the sheet, and with the other hand, he pulls up the patient's gown. He is careful to keep the genital area covered. He lifts the dressing covering the wound, causing the patient to flinch. The wound is short and vertically oriented in the midline of the abdomen. It begins below the navel and ends above the pubis. Evenly spaced steel staples run the length of the wound. In between the staples are a few crusts of dried blood. After a brief inspection, Dr. Jones tamps the loosened dressing back down against the patient's skin.

He declaims, "Looks good. The nurses will take care of the dressing for you. I'm going to try starting you on a diet. If that goes well, home soon."

"OK, Doctor."

The visit is fast and leaves the patient slightly bewildered. Dr. Jones is in the hospital corridor before the patient has a chance to ask questions. He glances at his watch. When he sees the time, he thinks, *got to get moving*. He hurriedly visits the next patient.

Doctor and patient exchange a few words. Satisfied the patient is recovering well, Dr. Jones briskly walks out of the room. He stops when he gets to the elevators that will take him from the fifth floor to the main level of the hospital. He waits impatiently for the elevator to arrive. A food cart appears pushed by a dietary worker, then a bed pushed by two nurses. In the bed is a withered elderly man. The man is burrowed down in the mattress. A plastic line dangles from the patient's neck and connects to an IV stand with an IV pump. The alarm on the IV pump beeps steadily. One of the nurses guides the IV stand with her right hand. Her left hand rests against the headboard of the bed. She leans her body forward as she pushes the heavy bed. An oxygen tank is lying in the bed with the patient. A hose runs from the nozzle on the oxygen tank to a mask over the patient's nose and mouth. Still the elevator doesn't come.

"Crap," Dr. Jones mutters and bolts for the stairwell.

Descending the stairs, Dr. Jones passes a hospitalist going in the opposite direction. The hospitalist pauses in his ascent when he sees Dr. Jones.

"Dan, I have a patient I want you to see. She came in last night, belly pain. Gynecology is seeing her too. I don't think it is appendicitis, but I want your opinion."

"What's her name? Is she on my list?" Dr. Jones says, temporarily forgetting there was only one new patient on his list.

"Michelle or Micelle—something close to that. She's on the third floor. I just wrote the consult. You'll be getting called about it soon."

"OK, I'll see her this afternoon. I have to get across town for a case right now."

Dr. Jones bounds down the stairs. In the main floor doctor's lounge, he gets his jacket and a cup of coffee. He exits the hospital and goes to his car in the doctor's parking lot. The car's interior is cold. The morning chill has not dissipated. He cranks up the heat and turns on the radio.

Leaving the parking lot, he passes Dr. Roice. Dr. Roice is driving a black Mercedes-Benz SLS Roadster. The Roadster is slowly easing into the parking lot. Following tacit doctor protocol, they lock eyes and gesture politely to each other. Dr. Jones, who is in a hurry, thinks of an impolite gesture he'd like to make.

A line of traffic is waiting to exit onto the highway Dr. Jones plans to take to get to the other hospital. He looks at the clock on the dashboard panel: 10:25 a.m. He is going to be late.

When Dr. Jones arrives at the operating room reception desk, he is still in his jacket. His white hair is askew, making him look a little like Dr. Einstein. He is not panting, but his chest heaves as if he may have been panting only moments before.

"OK, Jane. Here and ready to work. Let's get going," he says to the clerk.

Jane looks at him laconically and says, "Your case got bumped. Didn't you know? Your OR team went to do a stat C-section."

"What?" Dr. Jones throws up his hands. "Did anyone tell my patient?"

"I don't know. You can check with the holding room."

"Thanks," Dr. Jones says, grimacing.

Dr. Jones speaks with the patient and the patient's family in the surgical holding area. He sympathetically explains the cause of the delay. They receive the unpleasant news with surprising graciousness. Dr. Jones is relieved to avoid the uproar the delay might have caused. Quietly, he tells the holding room nurse to call him when the patient is ready to be moved to the operating room.

An hour passes, during which time Dr. Jones has rounded on his inpatients. By 11:50 a.m., Dr. Jones wonders why he hasn't heard anything from the operating room about starting his case.

When he calls the operating room receptionist, he learns the C-section is taking much longer than predicted. The baby was fine, but the mother was having unusually heavy postpartum uterine bleeding. Apparently the obstetrician had just succeeded in getting hemostasis and had started to close the wound. The receptionist thinks Dr. Jones may be able to start his case around 1:00 p.m.

III

AFTERNOON AND NIGHT

Impatiently waiting for a surgical team to become available, Dr. Jones goes to the locker room to change from his street clothes into the light blue scrubs he will wear during surgery. The scrubs are sized small, medium, large, extra large, XXL, and XXXL. They are sorted on the shelves accordingly. There is a tall stack of small scrubs, a shorter stack of medium scrubs, and only a stray pant or shirt left in the other sizes. Dr. Jones squeezes into a medium pant and dons the last large shirt. The scrubs are soft and comfortable from numerous washings. In a different context, they could be baggy old pajamas.

The phone in the locker room rings. When Dr. Jones answers the phone, he is told the C-section is finished, but the surgical team needs to go to lunch before starting his case. While that team is at lunch, someone else will set up room four for the gallbladder surgery. A reasonable plan since OR personnel arrive to work at 6:30 a.m. Despite this, Dr. Jones thinks, *more delay, day going downhill.*

He goes to the main doctor's lounge to get lunch. The hospital provides assorted snacks and food for the physicians. A refrigerator in the lounge is stocked with juices, water, and sodas. A second refrigerator has cold sandwiches, a few soups, and some distressed-looking salads. A bowl of fruit, ranging in quality from nearly fresh to nearly spoiled, sits on a table. The sandwiches, mostly limp, are made with damp, several-days-old bread. The microwave provided for warming the sandwiches, though serviceable, improves taste and appeal only slightly. The snacks, are commercially packaged, single-portion chips, peanut butter crackers, and cookies.

Dr. Jones warms a turkey-and-cheese sandwich. The sandwich, a bag of chips, and a soda comprise his lunch. While he is eating, other physicians pass in and out of the lounge. A television in the lounge is tuned to a cable news station. The droning of the host creates continuous background noise. Slowly, Dr. Jones becomes aware of the news segment about an ongoing meteor shower.

"For you astronomy buffs, the Leonids meteor shower that began earlier this week will peak tomorrow morning between the hours of midnight and six a.m.," the television announcer says. "During that time, thousands of tiny particles will enter the Earth's atmosphere and combust. Some of the larger particles will cause the streaks of light we often call shooting stars. Observers can hope to see as many as ten to twenty meteors per hour if conditions are favorable. A cloudless night is predicted, which should be ideal for viewing. The meteors will appear high in the sky early, then near the horizon closer to daylight."

The door to the doctor's lounge opens. An attractive, middle-aged brunette clerk from the hospital's Medical Records Department sashays into the room.

When she sees Dr. Jones eating his soggy turkey sandwich, she exclaims with false coquetry, "Ooh, my favorite doctor! I have been missing you in Medical Records."

She dashes out of the room. She returns a moment later carrying an inch-thick stack of papers held together by a single thick rubber band.

"Dr. Jones, I just need you to answer this one coding question. We can't finalize this patient's chart until you do."

She hands the papers to Dr. Jones, who delicately places the partially eaten sandwich on a napkin and then wipes his hands with another napkin before taking the papers. The patient, whose name, John Smith, appears at the bottom right-hand corner of each sheet of paper, is vaguely familiar to the doctor. The coding question is quite familiar. The question he reads is, "Was debridement excisional or nonexcisional?"

Debridement is the surgical term for cleansing a wound of decaying tissue. The technique of debridement can be chemical or mechanical. Mechanical debridement includes a variety of energy sources, which may include electricity, vibration, light (laser), or friction. The most common method is decidedly low tech. The devices Dr. Jones typically uses are scalpel and scissors.

"Kathy, he got better," Dr. Jones says wearily. "Does this really matter? He was discharged two months ago anyway."

She glowers at him imperiously. "It most certainly does matter! What's the matter with you? If you don't fill that out, you know you will be on suspension."

This is a threat to Dr. Jones. If he doesn't fill in his response she will tell the Hospital Administration Office to suspend his operating and admission privileges.

"Uh huh. And who is going to take call on Friday night?" he challenges.

Exasperated, he scrawls "EXCISIONAL!" across the blank space on the paper below the question with the date, time, and his signature.

"There, wasn't that easy?" Kathy says smugly. "You doctors!" She flounces out of the room.

Dr. Jones's pager goes off, emitting a shrill, high-pitched repetitive note. He involuntarily cringes, like a lab animal in some maleficent, behavior-conditioning experiment. *Now what?*

The number displayed on the pager is the operating room reception desk. When he answers the page, the receptionist tells him his patient is being put to sleep in operating room four. They are ready for him at last.

After putting on shoe covers and a surgical cap, Dr. Jones marches through the operating room. He stops in front of the scrub sink located outside operating room four. He peers into the operating room through the rectangular window above the sink. He sees the patient has been intubated, and her abdomen has been prepped with an orange surgical cleansing solution.

Satisfied the patient is, indeed, ready for surgery, he ties on his customary face mask and washes his hands and forearms with the astringent surgical soap. Arms dripping with soapy water, he enters the operating room and makes a rapid mental survey. He likes the team he has been given. Beneath his surgical mask, he smiles. The pupils of his brown eyes dilate slightly; the lateral angle where the upper and lower lids join crinkles.

The operating room environment is peculiar due to the absence of the visual cues normally used to infer mood or nuance of language. Hair and facial features are almost completely obscured by masks and caps. Bodies are covered in formless gowns. Operating room personnel become adept at interpreting the meaning of muffled voice, posture, and slight changes in the narrow strip of face extending from the middle of the forehead to the bridge of the nose. The staff in the room intuitively senses the doctor's demeanor.

"Welcome, Dr. Jones, to room four," the circulating OR nurse says expansively. "You've been waiting awhile. Sorry about that. We're glad you're here now."

Even though he is pleased to get the case started, he is not quite over his annoyance that his case, out of several possible candidates, was the one bumped for the C-section.

He chooses to ignore the nurse's comment and says to no one in particular, "All right. Let's get going."

The procedure, cholecystectomy (gallbladder removal), is the most commonly performed procedure in Dr. Jones's surgical repertoire. Although each procedure requires vigilance, this patient's gallbladder disease is not complicated. There is only a span of eight or ten minutes that requires Dr. Jones to focus intently. The critical time interval includes identifying and clipping the drainage tube from the gallbladder and controlling the blood supply to the gallbladder.

At the precise critical moment, Dr. Jones's pager goes off. He stops what he is doing and stands straighter.

"Pam," he says to the circulating nurse who is working the room, "can you get my pager and answer that?"

The nurse reaches inside his sterile gown and fumbles to free the pager from where it is attached to his scrub pants. When she has it securely in her grasp, she reads the number on the display.

"Three nine eight oh."

"That's third floor at the other hospital," Dr. Jones says. "Go ahead and call them."

He goes back to clipping the artery to the gallbladder. The nurse calls the number from the phone on the wall in the operating room.

After some conversation with the person on the other end of the connection, she says, "Dr. Jones, you have a consult on the third floor to rule out appendicitis. The patient's name is Micelle."

This is the patient the hospitalist had talked to Dr. Jones about in the stairwell when he was leaving the hospital.

"I know, I know," Dr. Jones says with rising annoyance. "Tell them to put her on my list, and I'll get to her when I can."

Three hours have passed since he first heard about the consult from the hospitalist. Almost as soon as the nurse hangs up the phone, the pager goes off again. Dr. Jones doesn't look up this time.

"Answer that."

The nurse dials a different number. Again there is some conversation.

"Dr. Jones, it's the ED here. They want to talk with you about a patient."

Dr. Jones shrugs his shoulders and shuffles his feet.

"All right. Put them on the speakerphone."

Dr. Jones keeps working.

"Hello, this is Dr. Reese in the ED."

The speakerphone makes it sound like Dr. Reese is far away, on another continent maybe.

"Go ahead. I can hear you," Dr. Jones says.

"Hey, sorry to disturb you in surgery. I just need your opinion about something. I have this patient with abdominal pain, no fever, no white count, but here is the tricky thing...the ultrasound shows a stone in the neck of the gallbladder."

"Any fluid around the gallbladder?" Dr. Jones asks.

"No."

Dr. Jones looks into the eyes of the scrub technician who is passing instruments for him. His eyelids open wider so the white sclera around the eye is more visible. She senses his frustration.

"Sounds like biliary colic," he says. "Give him something good for pain. Tell him he needs to see a surgeon soon and arrange for outpatient cholecystectomy. Not an emergency, but something he should do soon."

"OK. Thanks. I just hadn't seen that before."

The speakerphone cuts off.

Dr. Jones looks around the room and says disdainfully, "Not tricky. They teach us that in the first year of training."

The rest of the surgery is completed without incident.

Dr. Jones goes to the surgeon's lounge to dictate the operative note and to write the patient's postoperative orders. The patient goes to the post anesthesia care unit (PACU), formerly known as the recovery room. When he is finished with charting, Dr. Jones takes the patient record to the PACU. This is typically a perfunctory obligatory stop before leaving the OR area entirely. In this instance, his eyes brighten when he sees one of his favorite nurses is recovering his patient. Sarah is demure, petite, and youthful. She is gentle with and considerate of patients. With the medical staff, especially the male medical staff, she has an enticing good humor. Her banter is often amusingly self-deprecating. Dr. Jones knows from operating room gossip that she and her husband separated over the past year. She has five children, all under the age of six. They are under her care most of the time. Not surprisingly, she has lost weight. Dr. Jones flops the chart on the bed table behind her loudly enough to distract her from the patient.

"Hey, you've lost some weight," he remarks. "You're going to need some new clothes."

She smiles and shakes her head. "A smaller scrub top anyway," she says. "Never comes off where you want. At least not for us."

"Be glad. At my age, weight doesn't come off at all. Bet some guys will be chasing you now."

She smiles a second time, flattered he might really think that.

"Patient is doing well, thank you." She changes the topic and turns her back to the doctor while she checks the IV that drips a clear fluid in the patient's arm.

"Great. I might see you later. I'm on call tonight, you know," he says ambiguously.

"Heard that. You take care."

Dr. Jones gets to his car and begins the drive back to the first hospital where he hopes to see the consult and finish what is left of his rounds. The shoulder of the on ramp to the highway is dotted with orange, diamond-shaped signs warning of roadwork ahead. He merges onto the highway where cars are traveling five to ten miles per hour above the posted speed limit. The highway median and shoulder are lined with trapezoidal, steel-reinforced concrete crash barriers. Except for the unevenly spaced orange-and-white-ringed barrels, the concrete barriers extend for miles. A sign planted on the edge of what remains of the highway shoulder and towering over the concrete barrier warns, "Lane Shift Ahead."

When Dr. Jones's car crests a small rise in the road, there appears an expanse of freshly graded and leveled reddish brown earth. The landscape is dotted with hydraulic excavators, track-type tractors, cranes, and graders. Drivers, including Dr. Jones, are distracted by the magnitude of the construction. Suddenly, crazily, the lane shifts sharply right. Dr. Jones snaps his attention back to the highway. The speed of the traffic abruptly drops, cars veer right, brakes screech, some tires smoke. Dr. Jones's pager beeps. With one hand, he wrestles the pager out of the carrying case clipped to his belt. On the pager display, he recognizes the number of the hospital switchboard operator. The text alert on his cell phone chimes musically.

He drops the pager on the passenger seat and picks the cell phone out of the driver's side door pocket. The text message is from his daughter. With his thumb, he opens the message: "Dad, did you send the check for the band trip? (smiley-face emoticon)" Ahead, traffic is merging onto the highway from a major thoroughfare. Dr. Jones drops the phone back in the door pocket. He checks in the mirror to see if the left lane is open so he can safely move over away from the merging cars. Vehicles are flying by in the left lane, accelerating again after having slowed for the lane shift. Dr. Jones has to slow his car even more. A driver trying to merge honks at him and gives him the finger. His pager beeps stridently. He glances at the passenger seat and sees that the pager has slipped off the seat and fallen between the seat and the passenger door.

At the exit for the hospital, he leaves the highway. On the exit ramp, he is stopped in a line of cars waiting to turn left onto Commerce Street. He takes a relieved breath, lurches across the passenger seat, and grabs the pager. He looks at the message display and realizes the page was the hospital switchboard operator paging him a second time. He puts the pager back in the carrying case and calls the switchboard. The stoplight changes to green. He turns left across the intersection. He is only a mile or two from his destination, the hospital.

"Operator, this is Dr. Jones. You paged?"

"Oh, yes, but she hung up. It was an outside call. I can ring it for you."

"Go ahead."

He hears the phone ringing.

A woman answers. "Hello?"

"This is Dr. Jones. Were you trying to reach the surgeon on call?"

The woman starts explaining rashly without preamble. "I had surgery Tuesday. I was sent home two days ago. Is it normal to still hurt?"

"What kind of surgery did you have?"

"A hernia at my belly button."

"It wouldn't be unusual to hurt a few days or even a week or two. Depends on the hernia."

"I need more pain pills. I'm out."

"Did you call your surgeon?"

"I called the office, but the voicemail said they were closed until Monday. The operator said you were on call for Dr. Smith."

"I am on call for Dr. Smith, but I don't know you or anything about your case. If you are hurting that badly, you will have to go to Urgent Care or the Emergency Department." Dr.

Jones continues driving while he talks.

"You can't call in a prescription?"

"It's not that I can't. I won't. I don't call in narcotic prescriptions for patients I don't know."

"What good is it for you to be on call? You're worthless!" Click.

Arriving at the hospital, Dr. Jones parks in the doctor's lot, which is empty because it is Friday afternoon. He enters the hospital through the side door staff entrance. In the hallway, he passes one of the hospital's assistant administrators leaving the hospital. The administrator walks hurriedly, pulling on and adjusting his sport jacket as he goes.

"Heading out for the weekend?" Dr. Jones asks.

"Yeah, have to get home. Wife has a dinner party scheduled for us tonight. Have a good weekend."

"You too."

Dr. Jones wends through the hospital corridors to the main bank of elevators. He takes an elevator to the third floor to see Sheila Micelle in room 316. Before going to her room, Dr. Jones reviews her medical record on the computer. She is twenty years old, single, smokes one pack of cigarettes a day, and occasionally drinks alcohol. She does not have any history of prior surgery or major medical illness. She has one child, and the delivery was vaginal. Her blood count on admission was slightly high. She hasn't been febrile since entering the hospital. The CT scan of her abdomen and pelvis obtained during her stay in the ED showed some pelvic fluid. Because contrast enhancement was not used for the study, the radiologist was not able to identify the source of the fluid.

When Dr. Jones enters the patient's room, he sees her boyfriend in bed spooning with her. The patient is clothed in a hospital gown. The boyfriend is wearing a purple T-shirt and jeans. The visible portion of his arms is inked with tattoos. His biceps bulge, even without flexing his arms. He looks askance at the doctor, slides out of the bed, and settles into the bedside chair. Dr. Jones introduces himself to the patient.

With his hand, he gently coaxes her to turn from her side onto her back. Her abdomen, he notices, is flat and taut. There is a circular astral tattoo around her navel. Dr. Jones lightly palpates her abdomen. He pushes a little deeper and more firmly when he gets to the right lower quadrant. She responds with a wince and a soft, deep groan. At the same time, she flexes her right hip and knee.

Dr. Jones looks at her earnestly and says, "Sheila, you have peritonitis, infection in the belly cavity. I am going to explore your abdomen. I think you have appendicitis, and the appendix may be ruptured."

The young man in the corner drops his head.

Sheila nods to the doctor and says quizzically, "Surgery? When?"

"Soon. I have a short case to do ahead of you. While I do that, the nurses will get you ready for surgery."

"OK. What did you say your name was?"

"Dr. Jones."

Dr. Jones notifies the operating room staff to add Sheila Micelle to the schedule for an open appendectomy to follow the drainage of abscess procedure.

An hour later, Dr. Jones is in the operating room with his scalpel poised above the outstretched arm of the anesthetized Mr. Carpen. The arm, extended near a right angle from the patient's body, has been prepped and sterilely draped. It rests on a large arm board, not unlike an ironing board. Dr. Jones sits on a chair positioned inside the angle made by the arm and body. The surgical assistant sits on a chair across from and facing Dr. Jones. The surgical technician, who will pass instruments during the case, stands at the end of the arm board beyond the reach of the patient's open hand. At the surgical technician's side is a sterile stand supporting a tray of instruments.

Dr. Jones uses his free hand to feel for the point of greatest tension along the patient's arm. At the exact point of maximum tension, he inscribes a small incision along the long axis of the arm. When the scalpel slices the skin, a fountain of milky white pus spews out of the arm. The arc of the fountain streams high above the arm, past the edge of the arm board, and splashes the surgical technician's shoe.

"Oh gross!" she yelps. "I just got these shoes to wear in the OR."

The assistant snatches the suction tip and aspirates the puddle of pus pooling at the patient's elbow.

"Sorry, I didn't see that coming," Dr. Jones says apologetically. "There is a lot of pus here."

He jams his finger under the skin and feels for the direction of the abscess cavity. When he is certain of the direction of the tract, he slices open the overlying skin. There is brisk oozing of blood and pus. The assistant suctions away the glop. Dr. Jones packs the wound with bulky gauze. After several minutes, he removes the bloody dressing and examines the wound. Most of the bleeding has stopped. He irrigates the wound thoroughly and packs it with a different kind of gauze. A gauze roll and then an elastic roll are wound circumferentially about the arm and over the packed wound. The entire procedure has taken less than thirty minutes. With the dressing securely in place, Dr. Jones leaves the OR. Cleaning up and readying the room for the next case are tasks for the other members of the surgical team.

In the interim, Dr. Jones tells the patient's enabling wife that he drained a half pint of pus out of her husband's arm. She doesn't show alarm or even surprise.

After dictating and writing the postoperative orders, Dr. Jones takes a small break. The surgical team is opening the supplies for the appendectomy. An orderly has gone to get Sheila Micelle and bring her to the surgical holding area. Dr. Jones eats a pack of cheese crackers and downs a cup of coffee. He slumps into a battered, overstuffed cushioned chair in the surgeon's lounge. He props his feet on the ottoman and lets his head fall back. On the flat-screen television mounted on the wall, a former sports star and a host are babbling about football. He dozes. A housekeeper enters the room to empty trash. He wills himself back to consciousness. The sportscasters are still babbling. He has dozed only a few minutes.

"Dr. Jones, prepping in room four," a clarion voice booms over the intercom.

"Coming," he says.

The water from the faucet where he scrubs is, as always, cold. He enters the operating room.

The surgical technician gives him a sterile hand towel, and he dries his hands and arms. He checks the clock on the wall. More than an hour has elapsed since he left the room after draining the abscess. The other members of the surgical team have been busy the whole time. They didn't get a break.

"Good turnover time," Dr. Jones says peevishly.

The tone betrays the meaning of his comment.

"Yeah, Mr. Carpen was hard to wake up," the operating room nurse says. "It took a lot of stuff to keep him asleep."

"Oh, it's anesthesia's fault then?" Dr. Jones chides.

"Yeah. That's right, isn't it, Dave?"

"Huh?" Dave, the anesthetist, hasn't been listening.

Sheila Micelle is a surgeon's vision of the ideal patient. She is slim and healthy. Asleep, her flat belly makes a trough between the crests of her bony hips. Dr. Jones makes a 2.5-cm incision in the skin at a site on the abdomen below which he knows the appendix should be located. He deftly splits the muscles and enters the abdominal cavity.

Thin, watery pus bubbles out from the incision. He inserts his index finger into the wound and wriggles it inside the abdomen. When he feels the appendix, he flips it up toward the wound. He clamps the appendix and draws it out of the abdomen. The appendix is swollen and covered with a thick, sticky exudate, but it is intact.

Dr. Jones's pager beeps. He asks the nurse circulating the room to take the pager and call the number displayed. She does. The page is from the fifth floor. A surgical patient, not his patient, has a rash. Dr. Jones orders Benadryl.

The appendectomy continues. Dr. Jones clips and ties the appendix. He sews up the wound. When he goes to the waiting room, he tells the boyfriend that Sheila has simple appendicitis. She will be fine and can probably be discharged tomorrow. The young man doesn't ask questions.

Instead, he stammers, "That's good then, real good."

Dr. Jones leaves the boyfriend sitting alone in a corner of the waiting room. A dusty Gideon's Bible lies on a table by the young man's elbow. The television in the room flickers banal images.

By the time Dr. Jones dictates the postoperative note, writes orders, and hand-delivers the chart to the post-anesthesia care unit, it is 9:10 p.m. Since there is no work pending, at least none of which he is aware, he decides to drive home. His first act upon getting into the car is to check his cell phone for messages. There aren't any.

Concerned, he texts Molly: "Home yet? Everything OK?"

She texts back: "Yes. Just home."

"Have you eaten?"

"Yes."

"OK. Good. On my way home."

The drive to his house takes twenty minutes on a quiet weekday evening. Because it is Friday evening, even after 9:00 p.m., there is traffic. The restaurant parking lots he passes are full. Cars are backed up waiting to turn into the multiplex cinema. He drives on.

When he gets home, Dr. Jones finds both children in the living room. Molly has the television tuned to a teen drama, which she doesn't seem to be watching. She is texting frequently, almost without pause. David has taken a side cushion from the couch and thrown it on the floor. He is lying half on, half off of the cushion. Dr. Jones stands at the threshold to the living room. From this position, he can see David is playing a game on his tablet that involves animation and some hopping or jumping anime.

"Hi, guys. What's up?"

"Nothing," Molly says, "Julie fighting with Bryan. I'm trying an intervention now."

Dr. Jones knows Julie is one of Molly's friends.

"Who is Bryan?" he asks.

"Her boyfriend. Sort of anyway. They've been out a couple of times."

"Oh, uh huh. David, did Molly get you something to eat?"

Dr. Jones is anxious to know that the children's basic needs have been satisfied.

"Yeah, I had a hot dog at the game."

"Was that enough? Are you hungry?"

"I'm OK, Dad."

"Who won the game?"

"We did."

"Oh! What was the score?"

"I don't know." David looks at Molly. "Molly, what was the score?"

"I don't know. We were ahead most of the time. I didn't watch the end. How is call going?"

"Not too bad since I'm here, right?" Dr. Jones lets out a feeble chuckle.

"Yeah, what I thought." Molly goes back to texting Julie.

Dr. Jones hasn't eaten anything since the crackers in the surgeon's lounge hours ago. He looks in the refrigerator. He spies a plastic container filled with leftover spaghetti with marinara sauce. He puts the container in the microwave and sets the cook time to two minutes. The microwave buzzes. The house phone rings. Dr. Jones picks up the receiver.

"Dr. Jones?" says the hospital operator. "Can I connect you to the fifth floor?"

"Sure," he says resignedly.

He hears the phone ringing the fifth floor and then, "Fifth floor, may I help you?"

"This is Dr. Jones. Somebody paged?"

"It was MaryAnn. I'll connect you."

"Oh, Dr. Jones, I'm calling about Mr. Carpen. There's a big spot of blood showing through his dressing."

"He's awake? Alert? Vital signs are good?"

"Oh yeah, I just thought you should know."

"OK, reinforce the dressing as needed then. He'll be all right."

"Thanks. Have a good night."

"Thanks. Bye."

Dr. Jones takes the spaghetti from the microwave and carries it into the living room. He sits on the couch opposite the side where David removed the cushion. He eats the spaghetti and tries to show some interest in the teen drama on the television. He puts the soiled dish on the end table, raises his feet, and places them on the couch where the missing cushion should be. Soon, his torso slumps and his head droops forward. Dreaming, he has the sensation of falling. A paroxysm of the muscles jerks him awake. *Hypnagogia,* he thinks.

"Kids, I'm going to try to get some sleep."

The children respond in near chorus, "All right, Dad. Night, Dad."

He shuffles up the stairs to his bedroom where he slips out of his clothes. The bed is a king. He lays the unfolded clothes gently at the foot of the bed opposite the side where he will be sleeping. He glides under the covers in only his boxers. He is asleep in seconds.

IV

MORNING AGAIN

The phone rings. He throws out his hand and fumbles with the receiver.

"Hello."

No response. He realizes he has the receiver upside down. After more fumbling, he orients the receiver correctly against his ear and face.

"Hello, this is Dr. Jones."

"Dr. Jones, this is the operator. I'll connect you to the Emergency Department."

"Emergency Department. May I help you?"

"This is Dr. Jones. You called?"

"Oh, yes, Doctor. Just a moment for Dr. Redrum."

"Hey, sorry to wake you man. Sam Redrum here. I have a little lady for you brought in by EMS. She can't say much due to a stroke two years ago. She is a resident at the Coughlin Home. You know, the rest home?"

"Yeah, I know it."

Dr. Jones eyes the clock on his nightstand. The fluorescent digital numerals show 12:18 a.m.

"I just got the fax report of the CT scan I ordered. The night reader says free air in the belly cavity with pelvic fluid and colon thickening, probable diverticulitis."

"OK, I'll take care of it. What room is she in?"

"Room twelve."

Dr. Jones thinks, *how appropriate.*

"Put the nurse on the phone."

He knows from the report the patient needs surgery due to a perforated intestine. He instructs the nurse to get consent for surgical exploration of the abdomen with probable colostomy, and to notify the operating room team.

He drags himself out of bed and pulls on the clothes stacked at the foot of the bed. He looks at his reflection in the bathroom mirror. Tufts of hair stick out from his scalp like rooster tails. *Can't go to the ED looking like the Joker.* He wets his hands under the faucet and runs them through his hair. *Better.*

He checks on the children. David is asleep in his bed. Molly is asleep on the couch. He turns off the television.

With hardly any traffic, the drive to the ED goes quickly. Once in the ED, he gathers the few pieces of paper that constitute the patient's chart. He bums a stethoscope from one of the nurses. The patient in room twelve lies on a stretcher on her back. Her torso is elevated some fifteen degrees above horizontal. Her distended abdomen makes a mound over her thorax. Her arms and legs, though normal in length, are spindly from muscle wasting. She resembles a beetle flipped on its back. He introduces himself to the patient.

She looks at him and says, "Me got to go."

The nurse taking care of the patient explains that the patient, Geneva Wilkins, has had a stroke. She has a type of expressive aphasia. She can understand and comprehend speech, but she can only say, "Me got to go." Dr. Jones nods, indicating understanding.

"Geneva, I'm going to examine you."

He listens to her heart and lungs with the stethoscope. He palpates her protuberant abdomen. Her eyes look at him imploringly.

"Me...got...to...go," she says with emphasis.

"Geneva, I have to operate. Your CT scan shows there is a hole in your intestines. You're not going to get better until I get the hole closed and wash out the contamination."

Geneva turns her head to the wall. After some minutes, she says, "Me got to go."

The nurse says Geneva's older sister is on her way to the hospital to give consent for surgery.

By 1:40 a.m., the patient is asleep, prepped, and draped in the operating room. Dr. Jones has changed into scrubs and had a fortifying cup of black coffee. The water at the sink where he scrubs prior to entering the operating room feels colder than ever. The combination of black coffee and cold water helps him focus but makes him irritable. There is gallows humor in the operating room.

"Nothing like a two a.m. party," the nurse anesthetist says. "Was anybody asleep?"

"Sleep? What's that?" another nurse says. "I've been up since six-thirty yesterday morning."

Dr. Jones looks at her and mentally confirms that she looks like she has been awake for twenty hours. She's not wearing makeup, and there are sunken, dark crescents under her eyes. He incises the patient's belly, and the pungent odor of stool suffuses the room. The suction cannula is placed in the abdominal cavity and slurps up the coffee-colored liquid. Periodically bits of partially digested vegetable matter clog the cannula. Dr. Jones carefully folds two 18 x 18 cm gauze pads and drapes them over the small intestine. Claire, the surgical assistant working from the side of the table opposite Dr. Jones places a large curved retractor against the folded sponges and pulls firmly upward. This displaces the small intestine from the pelvis and lower abdomen. With the small intestine out of the way, Dr. Jones readily identifies a hole in the sigmoid colon, the part of the large intestine that is the typical site of diverticular disease.

The situation calls for the Hartmann procedure. The operation, first introduced by French surgeon Henri Hartmann, consists of removing the damaged or diseased segment of the large intestine with closure of the intra-abdominal rectal remnant and forming a proximal colostomy. Due to the relative ease of performance and a low complication rate, this procedure is the *bon ami* of surgeons who find themselves up to their elbows in abdomens full of shit. Dr. Jones and his team perform the procedure by rote. Though familiar, the operation does not yield to haste. It is 3:16 a.m. when the nurse anesthetist charts in her log that surgery has finished.

Dr. Jones walks away from the operating table. He unties his surgical gown and throws it in a heap on top of the laundry hamper. He drops his surgical gloves in the red medical waste container. Simultaneously, the nurse anesthetist gives the drugs that will reverse the patient's anesthesia. The operating room nurses pull off the patient's drapes and bundle up the soiled instruments to send to sterile processing. There is a flurry of activity behind him as Dr. Jones exits the room.

In the hallway, he tears off his surgical mask with one hand and slides off his cap with the other. He drags his hands through his white hair, which has become oily over the course of the day and is flattened against his scalp from the light but continuous pressure of the cap and mask he had been wearing. He enters the surgical waiting room and updates Geneva's sister about the surgical findings and the patient's condition.

The sister, whom he had not met earlier, resembles the patient. She is short and stout, and dressed in black slacks and a white top with a round, matronly collar. Over her top she wears a black cardigan sweater. Below her thick legs and ankles, she wears canvas flats. Her hair is white and thin and puffy. She introduces the man sitting by her side as her pastor. His age is similar to her own. Her face tells of her worry. The pastor is calm, silent, and supportive. A single table lamp illuminates the room with a soft, yellow glow. Dr. Jones is aware of the presence of other bodies in the room slumbering in the dark umbra beyond the lamplight.

He sits on the edge of a chair facing Geneva's sister and the pastor. He leans forward, elbows resting on his knees. He holds his hands together, the fingers curling over his knuckles.

"The surgery went well," he says. "Geneva is doing well. Anesthesia is waking her up now, and she will be going to the recovery room shortly. She had an infection of the large intestine as expected. Diverticulitis. I know you might be worried about cancer. I don't suspect cancer, but of course, our pathologist will look at the specimen."

The pastor gently pats the sister's leg and says, "Mary, I told you she would be all right."

"Doctor, when will I be able to see my sister?" Mary asks.

"She'll be in recovery about an hour. Someone will call and let you know the room assignment. You can see her when she gets to her room."

"Let them know I will be waiting, Doctor. Pastor, you can go. Thank you for coming.

"Doctor, bless you," Mary continues. "My sister and I are the only ones left. I am not ready to give her up quite yet, but that is not up to me."

Dr. Jones rises from the chair and backs out of the room.

"Mary, we'll do the best we can for Geneva."

Dr. Jones goes to the surgeon's lounge where the prior evening he had dozed in front of the flat-screen television. He dictates the postoperative note and writes the postoperative orders. For a moment, he feels content. Call is almost finished. He has completed the last task he hopes for this call day.

He enters post-anesthesia care as the patient is being wheeled into the room on a gurney from the OR.

He smiles as he hears her say weakly, "Me got to go."

Yes, me got to go. Wordlessly, he drops the thin chart on the post-anesthesia care desk.

Leaving the hospital, he drives down empty residential streets lined with rows of dark houses. He waits at the stoplight before turning left on Commerce Street. On the side of the road opposite, he can see the glow of light from a small all-night diner. A few cars are clustered around the entrance. Through the diner windows he can clearly see customers, the straggling remnants of the night's uptown revelry.

The stoplight changes from red to green, and soon Dr. Jones is on the highway. Overhead is a pellucid sky. The myriad stars shine brightly.

Absentmindedly, Dr. Jones takes the route that delivers him to the cul-de-sac where his house looms. The car bumps into the driveway and begins the descent to the garage. A meteor streaks evanescently across the horizon.

He doesn't notice.

V

EPILOGUE

The practicing lifespan of a surgeon is thirty to thirty-five years from the end of training to retirement. During this time historically it has not been unusual for a surgeon to take call every third or fourth night. This is equivalent to eleven years on call. Changing aspects of healthcare are causing newly trained surgeons to seek employment models that limit exposure to call and allow for a more manageable lifestyle. The surprise is not that the current model of call is getting wobbly, but that it has functioned so well for so long.